Hot

Flourishes

Snippets of wisdom and whimsy
for menopausal women

Dawn Robinson

©2022 by Dawn Robinson

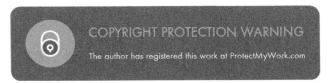

For Jeanne Day who taught me how to
embrace aging fearlessly and showed me the
possibility of climbing Munros in your eighties.

And for my lovely email subscribers who have read my
Midlife Flourishes over the years and
given me the encouragement to keep writing.
Thank-you.

A huge welcome to Hot Flourishes

 A huge welcome to Hot Flourishes and I'm so delighted you've joined me here.

We can all have those days when life feels a little out of control and crazy and this collection of snippets of wisdom and whimsy are for just those times.

They are the result of several years of regular Midlife Flourishes sent to my mailing list and posted on social media, written through the ups and downs of my own life and I hope you find them both comforting and inspiring.

You'll see that I've used both the words "midlife" and "menopause". In this book the words are interchangeable but if one makes more sense to you, obviously feel free to swop them around.

This book isn't particularly about the physical challenges of menopause but I do believe that our emotional and mental health have a huge impact on how we experience this time of life and so these aspects have been my focus here.

I strongly believe that when we regularly tap into our innate resilience and wisdom, we can emerge stronger and I hope that in some small way, this book helps you along this journey.

So are you sitting comfortably? Then let us begin...

Much love
Dawn x

Once upon a time, there was a princess who reached menopause and felt her life was a mess and she had turned into a wrinkly old frog.

Unfortunately, there was no handsome prince or fairy godmother to make it all better, so (as usual) she had to sort it out herself.

And then finally, she unleashed her own magic and realised how powerful and strong she had been all along (something she had never for one moment suspected as a young, dippy princess with a pretty smile).

And so she lived happily ever after creating her own perfectly wonderful life.

Today reclaim your sense of wonder.

For a world spinning around a sun.

For a new day and a gentle moment.

For your beating heart and a soft smile.

How could you live more adventurously?

I'm not talking about walking around the world, cycling across the country or paddling down the nearest river.

Although if these seem like great ideas to you, why not?

This is about taking a small step towards a dream you have.

Going somewhere different.

Meeting someone new.

Allowing yourself to be bolder.

Living adventurously, on your terms.

What if menopause were the interval between the two great Acts of life, Youth and Age?

What if it were a chance to refresh your make-up, take stock and recharge yourself for the most magnificent performance of your life?

Act 2 - when it's really time to show the audience what you're made of.

Act 1 was just the warm up act!

Menopausal Wonder Woman pants may be slightly larger and have more stretch in them.

And you're an amazing woman who's capable of very great things so don't be afraid to wear them more often.

What if you could step into the future, into your vibrant eighty year old self?

As this incredible, wise woman, what would you lovingly say to your very youthful menopausal self?

What advice would you offer?

Which dreams would you encourage yourself to reach for?

From the perspective of an eighty year old there's masses of time and energy left for you to create an amazing present and future.

Remember the quality of your life doesn't come from the numbers when you weigh yourself, the amount of money you have in the bank or the likes you have on your social media posts.

It comes from what's going on inside your head.

Which thoughts you pay attention to.

Always.

Rules for life number 386

The solution to that problem that's been haunting you for days is never going to turn up whilst you're anxiously ruminating over numerous options or forcing yourself to think of the answer.

It'll come unannounced when you're out dancing on those tables, skydiving out of that plane or quietly watching the sun go down.

Relax.

And allow the answers to all problems to arrive in their own time.

The truth about scary thoughts..

Have a scary thought

Accept it as the truth

Get scared

Listen to another scary thought

Accept that as the truth too

Get even more scared

Listen to yet more scary thoughts

doom
and
gloom

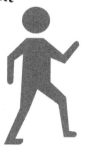

Have a scary thought

See it as impersonal
and not important

Carry on with life

When life feels overwhelming or a struggle, don't be afraid to sit gently with all your feelings and really feel them.

Trust that the wisdom of your body that knows how to heal a cut on your finger, also looks after your mind and your heart (even if sometimes I'll admit, it feels as if all hell is breaking loose!!!).

When was the last time you did something fun?

And I'm not talking about the grown-up, serious kind.

But daft fun, silly fun?

Popping bubble wrap (my personal favourite), jumping in a puddle, catching a flying leaf.

All possibilities for today as well as walking the dog, chairing that very important meeting and balancing the finances.

**Effortless transformation or change
is merely a thought or insight away.**

Forcing ourselves to change or
struggling with willpower, not required.

Seeing something different, telling
ourselves a new story is all that we
need.

Taking our thoughts, all of them, with a pinch of salt, treating each of them lightly is the best way to inhibit any tendencies they may have to take themselves too seriously and turn into thought divas.

No matter what is going on in your life and the ups and downs you're faced with, the potential for wellbeing is always yours.

Never think for a moment that it's deserted you.

Wellbeing is who you are.

How amazing is it that someone else put the rubbish bin out last night!

How incredible that my daughter didn't need to be prompted eighty-five times to get ready for school this morning!

The delivery man turned up on time, the new furniture was put together without frayed tempers and there was a square of chocolate left in my super, secret, hidden stash.

Even in the everyday, the humdrum and domestic, there are miracles aplenty, every day.

When we're feeling stressed, I can guarantee we're caught up in the overthinking mind.

Taken from Ditch Your Midlife Stress From the Inside Out: Dawn Robinson.

In any situation that seems scary, tricky or challenging, all we ever need to do is what we feel moved to do in that moment.

That's it.

No overthinking, getting ourselves caught up in knickers-in-a-twist, thought knots or internal debating required.

Thoughts will be passing through your mind all day long.

It might be interesting to note which ones you are holding onto.

Remember, you can always choose which ones you pay attention to and which ones you just allow to gently pass on by.

**Life can guide us every step of the
way but we have to be looking to see
the directions.**

We have to be quiet enough to listen to
the whispers.

It's not complicated and it's not tricky.

And there's an incredible joy to be
found in loosening our grip on
controlling life.

Enabling everything to become so
much easier.

Menopause.

**Not a time to be creeping
apologetically through life.**

A time to be seen, to be heard and to
share your many gifts whatever your
fears and your doubts.

There is always the possibility for something new, a fresh start.

Never underestimate your capacity for change and seeing your life differently.

And this can happen in a heartbeat.

Our minds contain a time machine.

Taking us forwards or backwards
through the years whenever we
choose.

And yet a wise woman knows that
keeping the time machine in it's box
(for the most part) is when our lives
are lived most fully and happily.

We live our lives in stress because of thoughts and emotions that have nothing to do with right here, right now but are rooted in thoughts about the past or the future.

Taken from Ditch Your Midlife Stress From the Inside Out: Dawn Robinson.

Are you going to wait until your life is blown onto a different course by the full force of storm winds?

Or is your mind quiet enough to hear the delicate whisperings of that knowing you have inside that's guiding you gently moment by moment?

How to deal with stress

Previously...

A new way of being.

- ☑ Meditation
- ☑ Visualisation
- ☑ CBT
- ☑ Spa days away
- ☑ Exercise
- ☑ Slump on sofa
- ☑ Drink, eat, spend too much

- ☑ Understand where our experience of stress is really coming from (hint - it's coming from our thinking).

- ☑ Go and make a cup of tea/ hot milky drink

- ☑ Get on with our life

Some women love my Hot Flourishes. Happy dance!

And others think they're rubbish.

I know bonkers isn't it?

But regardless, I'll keep on writing them because this is what I know to be true.....

Some people will love what you do and think you're amazing.

Others will turn up their noses and sneer.

But keep on creating, my lovely, whether it's a herb garden, a novel about running away to the circus or a knitted hat.

Whatever's in your heart to bring into the world do it, because not to do so would set off all the creation fairies crying into their hankies with sorrow.

And trust me, we really don't want to let that happen.

Never, ever underestimate your power to make this beautiful world a better place.

Even when it seems as if we have such a small part to play.

Each of us, in so many ways, can spin webs of love, hope and inspiration.

How to deal with problems.

Do what needs to be done, NOW, in this moment.

Trust your own intuition and get expert help when that feels like the right thing to do.

Don't overthink it and ignore the looking-into-a-crystal-ball-this-is-going-to-be-awful thinking.

And I know that I've said this before, but trust yourself.

When discouragement haunts you, remember that we're not in charge of the timescale of our success.

Nor can we ever know how vital each tiny setback is in the journey to our goals.

When we can accept these truths, hope and determination are ours once more.

There can be such joy in the simple moments.

The falling of a leaf, sun through a window, the sound of rain, the comfort of an embrace.

Allow the chatter of your mind to dissolve and enjoy each tiny, perfect sliver of your life.

Give yourself permission to feel what you feel.

The feelings we embrace and those we resist are all part of the glorious experience of being human.

Every one of them.

And the more we allow any feelings (even the nasty, pesky ones) to just be, the easier they naturally flow.

Trying to rush decisions, making them ahead of time, is as pointless as trying to choreograph an entire discussion with a friend three weeks in advance.

Taken from Ditch Your Midlife Stress From the Inside Out: Dawn Robinson.

There will always be burdens to carry, ups and seemingly endless downs.

Life was ever so.

Be gentle.

Treat yourself with compassion.

Allow the cycles of life to play out in your life.

When you have energy, dance, sing and take the inspired steps of action.

When you are weary, retreat and rest.

It can be as simple as this.

**Never doubt your own amazingness
even when self-doubt seems to hold
you in its grasp.**

Don't argue that your life is normal,
that extraordinary isn't for you.

You are brilliant in your own way.

Taking steps to improve our life is part of our growth.

But remember to be ok with what is, right now, in this moment.

In the words of one of my favourite-ever programmes, "Resistance is futile."

Anxious? Stressed?

Grappling with these emotions never interferes with our innate capacity for mental and emotional health and wellbeing.

Never, ever.

Doing less isn't always easy.

We set such store on being busy, productive, on getting things done.

But if we think about it, our most precious, beautiful memories are when we are just being with others, in nature, or enjoying our solitude.

It might be worth pausing to create more of these delicious memories once in a while.

Those thoughts that drift through your mind - the ones that delight, entertain, frighten, frustrate and shatter your peace.

They are like clouds drifting across the sky.

They are not you.

You are something much more.

You are not your thoughts.

All that is ever required of us is to be fully present so that we are awake and aware.

Awake to who we really are, aware of our true potential and brilliance and open and ready, for whatever life might bring.

Taken from Ditch Your Midlife Stress From the Inside Out: Dawn Robinson.

Every day, each moment has the potential to be lived fully.

Collapsing into a heap, working in a very grown-up way, embarrassing mum dancing, sobbing until our nose runs, snorting with laughter.

Let's throw ourselves into all of it fully and completely.

Trust yourself.

Have faith in all that you are and take
a deep, calm, slow breath.

You can handle it.

All of it.

Even this.

There's a quirk of inner wisdom that we often overlook when we browse through the How to Tap into Your Own Guidance handbook.

It gets activated in the present moment.

What do I need to do now? - works brilliantly.

What do I need to do in three weeks time? Any answers are going to be a bit more dodgy.

The road towards our dreams and goals is never a straight line.

So often, it's a meandering track with many twists and turns.

At times, it can feel as if we're retracing old steps.

But stay on the path, keep looking ahead and keep putting one foot in front of the other.

Menopause can feel very tough at times.

Get help if you need to, seek advice.

But know this.

Your body has a powerful innate wisdom and Mother Nature hasn't abandoned you.

In a low mood

Accurate and helpful thoughts

Overly pessimistic and inaccurate thoughts

In a good mood

Overly pessimistic and inaccurate thoughts

Accurate and helpful thoughts

Disappointment.

Part of life's flow of ups and downs, the rhythm of living or something to battle?

You decide.

Treat yourself with the utmost care.

Throughout every emotion, with each passing thought, hold yourself gently.

You are exquisite, beautiful and very, very precious.

Not broken, weak or damaged but still in need of tender care, nevertheless.

Step lightly into your dreams.

There's no need to carry the extra bucket loads of overthinking, doubts and fears.

Hold the question "What's my next step?" gently in your mind and listen for the answer.

Then take action.

Call it fate if you will or destiny but despite our best intentions, life has paths for each of us that are above and beyond that which we see for ourselves.

They show up in the unexpected twists of fate, the unforeseen happy co-incidences or the out of the blue opportunities.

Taken from Ditch Your Midlife Stress From the Inside Out: Dawn Robinson.

There comes a time in every life when we start to question who we are and where we're going.

Whether we listen to the soft murmurings or wait until our heart, body and soul are crying out in desperation for change is the difference between a midlife crisis and a midlife evolution.

**Little Miss Muffet sat on a tuffet,
eating her curds and whey.**

Along came a spider who sat down
beside her...............

And because Miss Muffet was fifty-six
and not afraid of wriggly creatures
anymore, the two sat happily together
eating their breakfast.

How far could you go in your midlife?

How much could you expand your idea of what you're capable of?

Now double it, triple it - push it to its extreme.

And if that feels scary, just keep breathing.

You know those dreams that have been whispering in your ear?

Now's the perfect time to go for them.

Where can you sit on a beautiful morning to listen to birdsong?

What if you took a moment at midday to feel a soft breeze on your cheek?

Why not spend some time gazing up at the stars?

You may feel that time is running out, that life is rushing past you, the years are speeding up.

But chill, my lover (as we say in Devon).

There's still plenty of time to start something new, create something different.

Time for fun and experience and joy.

There's masses of time for life.

Trying to control what thoughts we have is an impossibility.

Attempting to change our thoughts is a futile battle.

But making choices about which ones we focus on - that's where the freedom lies.

You know there are things you find easy.

Things that others marvel at.

So what if it was all easy?

Come on now, I don't want to hear those "yes, buts......" because if it really is that difficult, do something else, find another way.

But most of all, give yourself a break and allow as much to be as super easy peasy as possible.

It's time to say goodbye to the complicated and embrace simplicity.

I see you.

I know who you really are.

Not "little you" tied up with the concerns of the day.

But the "expansive you".

The one who is magnificent and powerful and perfectly marvelous.

Now see who you really are.

A quiet, spacious mind is our natural default.

When we stop living frantically, rushing around, filling our mind with worries and stresses, the mental equivalent of junk food, it naturally settles by itself.

There is nothing we have to do to find this state, no skill we need to learn, master or develop.

Taken from Ditch Your Midlife Stress From the Inside Out: Dawn Robinson.

The whole self-improvement lark is actually leading you up a false trail.

You want to know why?

Well you're already as self-improved as you ever could be.

That's not to say that you can't have a little extra project on the side to deal with those habits/ get fit/ have more fun, but fundamentally you're perfection already, I'd say!

Long ago, when we were very young,
we made up stories about our
limitations, our inadequacies.

And gradually, we started to believe
our stories were The Truth.

But believing these tales, made us
miserable, kept us small and squashed.

It's time to ditch these old fantasy
tales.

Time to find more expansive stories
and a bigger Truth.

Not everything we desire comes to us.

Not everything we wish for, will be ours.

But inside us is a deep well of creativity and inspiration that we can turn to whenever we choose to make sure as hell that we stack the dreams-come-true odds in our favour.

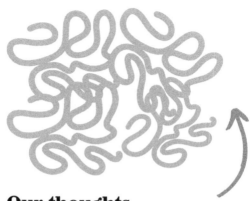

Our thoughts when we're overwhelmed

Our thoughts when we're calm and our mind is quiet

We don't have to know how we're going to achieve our dreams.

We never need to anticipate the problems that lie ahead or the extent of what will be required of us along the way.

We just have to know that it's our dream.

We only need to take the first tiny step and know the step after that will then show itself.

That's all that's required of us.

To move forward, carefully, in a mad dash or however way we choose and to put up a very disrespectful two fingers to the analysis, overthinking and doubt!

Menopause.

Perplexing?

An opportunity for change and growth?

Painful. exhilarating, tiresome, joyful?

Whatever it means to you, it's also a gift.

It's a time of life that has been denied to so many women.

It's ours to make of what we choose and to cherish.

When I'm seventy-two I'd like to win Ice Skater Of The Year award

(a special award for people who started skating in their late forties and have never shown an inkling of talent whatsoever but have carried on regardless).

When I'm eighty-eight I'd love to take up a new sport – possibly extreme knitting on the top of a mountain. I'll take a picnic which we can share if you'd like to join me.

What would you wish for yourself in the future?

No matter what our age, we've always got to keep on dreaming and planning and now is the time to start preparing to make these dreams for our old age, a reality.

Once we start to tap into this deep inner knowing or internal wisdom, it becomes obvious that we do know what needs to be done.

Doors need to be slammed shut on doomed love matches, gooey chocolate cakes need to be left on supermarket shelves and tickets for exciting new adventures need to be booked.

Taken from Ditch Your Midlife Stress From the Inside Out: Dawn Robinson.

Midlife.

A time to be bold and flamboyant.

A time to take brave steps forward and kick midlife invisibility up into the stratosphere.

A time for laughter, fun and making a difference.

Be it. Live it. Love it.

You're either living fully and embracing every opportunity and experience.

Or you're not.

Just saying!

Our feelings never remain static.

Even deep, turbulent feelings like rage or grief, have their time and, if we let them, will move through us.

Taken from Ditch Your Midlife Stress From the Inside Out: Dawn Robinson.

Time for the commercial break

 Are you a midlife, menopausal woman who seems to have misplaced her joy in living in the frantic busyness of life?
Struggling to calm down and enjoy the moment? Looking for a way of helping your body and your mind gently slow down and regain that feeling of inner serenity?

What you need is **The Hot Flourishes Relaxation** - a gently calming audio journey to soothe your body and mind.

The Hot Flourishes Relaxation the marvelously delectable, **FREE** guided meditation can be yours now.

Just scan the square thingy below or visit www.theflourishingmidlife.com/hotflourishes

I don't know when we start believing that the fun, crazy adventures, the deep loves and wild times are behind us.

But this is a MOMENTOUS mistake, (still an easy one to make I suppose!).

They're all there waiting for us now and in the future, if we choose.

It's all working out perfectly (although let's face it, it might not seem like it at the time).

Through every miniscule setback, every furrowed brow and tear of frustration shed, we need to hold onto this thought.

It will all come good.

Whilst none of the thoughts coming into our mind are under our control nor do we have to pay attention to them once they arrive either.

We don't have to accept them as The Truth and we certainly never have to view them as a reflection of who we are.

Taken from Ditch Your Midlife Stress From the Inside Out: Dawn Robinson.

Where to look to answers

Previously...

☑ Ask a friend

☑ Consult an expert

☑ Look at tea leaves

☑ Google it

☑ Ask the pub "expert"

☑ Youtube

A new way of being.

☑ Listen to our own innate wisdom

☑ Allow inspiration to come where and when it will and do what seems to make sense in the moment (might include any on left)

☑ Get on with life

Let's give a cheer for all us menopausal women juggling strange physical symptoms, wild moods, sudden rages, career, family, finances, lunch box preparation...

Makes me feel quite overcome thinking how much we all contribute, how much we give.

With so much love and respect for all you do, all that you are.

Your experience of life, the good, the bad, the tedious, the outrageous is never, ever coming from the outside world and circumstances (even though it can look pretty convincing).

It is always, always coming from your own thinking.

And even if this seems completely bonkers, there are no exceptions.

Sing a song of sixpence, a pocket full of rye.

Four and twenty blackbirds were baked in a pie.

When the pie was opened, the birds began to sing and the menopausal, brain fog distracted woman wondered what the heck had happened as she had intended to bake a chicken and ham pie and she must have got distracted.

Your biggest ever challenge is dealing with an analysing, critical mind that's always whining and whirring, on and on and on.

What you've got going for you is the mind that lies beneath all of this drama.

A place of stillness and calm where unending wisdom lies.

We think, but we are never, ever our thoughts.

No matter how beautiful or scary they are.

We're something separate from that, something greater.

We're the space in which these thoughts occur.

It doesn't really matter how close or how far we are from achieving that goal.

All we have to do is keep putting one foot in front of the other and carry on plodding because we never really know when life is going to give us a pair of wings to fly there faster.

Is there something you've always longed to do or experience?

It's time to give yourself permission to get on and do it.

Now. Today. No excuses.

Midlife.

Old enough to know who we really are.

Mature enough to recognise what needs to change, what's going to have to go and what's for keeps.

Young enough to try something new and exciting.

Today is World Walking on Grass Day (ok so I might have made that up!).

Find time to wiggle your toes in grass and remind yourself how simple and uncomplicated pleasure can be.

Who are you?

Who is the real you?

Even now at forty, fifty, sixty and beyond, there's always the possibility of expanding and changing the answer to those questions.

Always room for change.

When you're in a situation you need to change, keep your senses and mind open for new or unusual solutions to come from other people, your day to day world, or things you hear or see.

Be ready to be amazed by how easy and straightforward the solution will seem.

Taken from Ditch Your Midlife Stress From the Inside Out: Dawn Robinson.

For when you need a little respite from older and wiser.

Find somewhere where you won't be disturbed and put on a song you loved in your twenties.

Dance wildly with abandon, (completely ignore the teenage daughter eye rolls) and enjoy.

How are you doing?

Isn't it funny how often we ask that?

As if our actions in the world were the most important part of us, as if who we are being were a secondary consideration.

You already have all the resilience, resourcefulness and strength you could ever need.

How do I know this?

Ah - I'm a midlife woman who's seen quite a bit of life and I know these things.

You've got this.

Dismiss the people who say "You can't, you're too old, it won't work", with a smile.

Don't give energy and attention to their doubts.

Nurture your relationships with the beautiful people who support, encourage and celebrate you.

They're the ones who see you as you truly are.

Only you know the answer to your problems.

Only you can turn to face the direction that's perfect for you in life and make the right choices.

It's all in your hands.

Believe in you.

Despite all the grand plans, the striving for and the hustling, the future is never quite what we imagine.

Maybe its time to set our goals, do what we can and then relax into wherever life takes us.

Ending any relationship can be tricky, especially with someone you've known your whole life.

Let's face it, Young You was lovely.

She was strong and beautiful but she did some pretty immature things, she made some crazy mistakes.

Mourn her passing by all means but another You will take her place.

Maybe her charms are less immediately obvious, her muscles less toned but she's got enough wisdom, insight and strength to blow your socks off.

Looking back of course I have regrets (you may have some too).

Bucket loads of them.

"If only I'd......"
"I wish I'd....."

But remember, throughout those years, we were always only ever doing the best we could at the time.

Are you rushing from one commitment to the next?

Is your life a high-speed train from morning open eyes to evening touch the pillow?

Allow there to be pauses in your day.

Give yourself brief precious moments to stop and breathe.

Turn your attention to your beautiful, hard-working body and feel its vitality and wonder.

As you look back over your life you might also notice how so often it's the difficult times in our lives that turn out in hindsight to be the catalyst for significant personal growth.

Taken from Ditch Your Midlife Stress From the Inside Out: Dawn Robinson.

How to solve any self esteem issue.

1. Stop looking outside yourself for reassurance and confirmation that you're doing ok.

2. Remind yourself that you've got this far, survived all you've been through and you're not a wibbly-wobbly wreck.

You've got all the inner resources, strength and knock-them over amazingness you could ever need, already.

3. Go out to play, have fun and get on with enjoying your life.

4. If you're like me you might have to repeat steps 1 - 3 on a regular basis but that's ok!

Our moods, stress and the accuracy of our perception

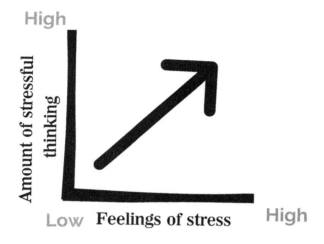

High

Amount of stressful thinking

Low Feelings of stress High

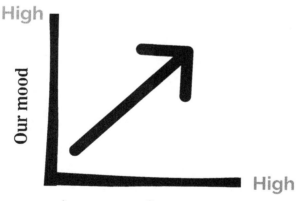

High

Our mood

High

Low Accuracy of our perception of the world

Have faith in all that you are and take a long, slow breath.

You can handle it.

All of it.

Is menopause leaving you feeling jaded?

Take a moment to look around, to listen, to engage your senses.

Step out of the half-dazed stupor of the busy, chatting mind.

And then you can rediscover the wonder and magic of this beautiful, incredible planet.

When you were a child, what did you want to be when you grew up?

Astronaut? Explorer? Dancer?

Me?

I wanted to be a fairy.

Midlife is the time to rekindle our youthful dreams.

Don't know about you but I'm off to buy myself a floaty skirt, a bit of sparkle and that must have fairy staple, a magic wand.

Sprinkling fairy dust on your wonderful dreams.

Humpty Dumpty sat on a wall, And all the King's horses and all the King's men, couldn't put Humpty together again.

So they sent in a middle-aged woman and she patched him up, soothed him with a hot chocolate and finally tucked him into bed because well, that's what we do.

We get stuff sorted!

Full of admiration for all that we do.

Menopause is the time to heal what needs to be healed.

In you.

In your life.

Once and for all.

When our mind is quieter, there's less internal chatter about our ability (or lack) of achieving our goals.

There's no inner debate taking place, no resistance and fear.

Just an awareness of the next step to take.

We see the distinction between what needs to be done and what's irrelevant time-wasting.

Taken from Ditch Your Midlife Stress From the Inside Out: Dawn Robinson.

Do you really want to shuffle through your midlife, tiptoeing politely so as not to disturb anyone?

Perhaps you might prefer to.....pull on those thigh-high suede boots, get out there and strut.

Be bold.

Dare to be seen and heard.

Feeling stuck?

Unsure of your next step?

Change your perspective for a while and just notice what fresh thinking comes to mind.

Remember, we're all perched on a planet that's rotating through space.

One of millions upon millions in endless universes.

And in a place so vast, there's always another option available lurking amongst those stars.

I woke up in such a foul mood this morning.

Everyone ran for cover.

Perhaps I should have used one of my 4683 ideas for mood enhancement.

But I didn't.

I just allowed it to be and eventually it moved on.

Healthy, cheery mood resumed and everyone crept out from their hiding places.

Such is the normal flow of our very human ups and downs - nothing we need to do about them other than watch them pass.

Midlife - perhaps it's a party.

Dress like it.

Put on the glitter and sparkle.

Or it could be a celebration.

Dance like it.

Follow the rhythm, flow and beat.

Or maybe a deep connection with old
and new friends.

Laugh long and deeply.

Make your midlife count.

Make it beautiful, joyous and glorious
in whichever way you chose.

There is never a moment when you're not the possessor of all the inner resources you'll ever need.

Confidence, resilience, a wealth of inspiration and creative ideas.

All there.

You just have to turn your attention from what's out there and look inside.

What could you do today that is so foot-tappingly wonderful that you set that warm glow inside alight!

How could you make someone else's day?

What can you do for yourself that creates a little joy?

When you think about it, it's not too difficult to change a mediocre day into one sprinkled with fun, happiness and a little dusting of magic.

Our moods are simply..........

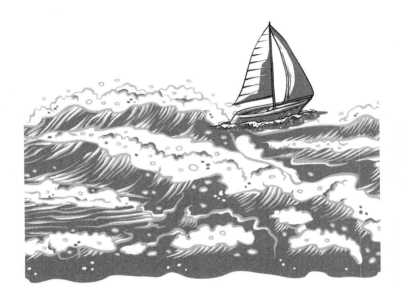

the ups and downs on the waves of life

What if change were easy?

No will power required, no internal struggles necessary, just effortless steps in the right direction.

You don't have to believe this or know it to be true.

Just allow the question to echo around your mind as you live each new day and keep your eyes peeled for the evidence.

Take a look at your hands.

Mine are starting to look weathered, to show my age.

Maybe yours do too.

But let's remember.

These hands however they look, dry tears, reach out to loved ones, write words to heal and create meals to nourish.

There are times in life when the road ahead is hidden.

Like walking through fog.

But we can always see a little ahead of us.

The next tiny step is always there.

And taking that one pace forward is all that's ever required.

Fallen into a midlife rut!

Do something new, something
incredibly daring and brave.

Or even something tiny and just on the
edge of scary.

Oh and don't forget to send me a
postcard about your adventures.

Stop all your fretting and worrying and analysing.

"But how?" I'm often asked.

Become aware of which direction your thoughts are taking you.

If you notice they're leading you down the train track of doom, just that one act of observing your thoughts rather than being caught in them is all that it takes.

Grappling with stress never interferes with our innate capacity for mental and emotional health and wellbeing.

At any moment, no matter our current level of joy or despair we always have the potential for new thought, different ways of being and a never-ending supply of creativity and inspiration that can transform us from wobbling disaster to self-assured, calm superheroine.

Taken from Ditch Your Midlife Stress From the Inside Out: Dawn Robinson.

The secret to living a life of menopausal ease.

1. Allow the mind to quieten.

2. Listen to the promptings of your soul.

3. Take action.

4. Repeat.

Setbacks and disappointments can momentarily make us forget how magnificent we really are.

Tears, stamping feet or miserable down-in-the-dumps pouts are all allowed and totally normal reactions to the frustrations of life.

Give yourself space for them.

But please, please, please, when you've had a little time to feel what you feel, get back out there and show us again, your wonderfulness.

The most freeing thing about midlife is realizing we're free to make up our own rules.

You're stressed, anxious, having a bad day.

How many thoughts per minute are you having?

Thirty-eight thousand, four hundred and two.

You're relaxed, calm, contentedly joyful.

How many thoughts per minute?

Four? Eight?

When you're having a bad day, just allow those thoughts to slow down and settle.

We all get caught up in the stories at some point.

Then at some point, we'll fall out of the illusions once more.

And this is just how it is.

It's all working out perfectly.

Psst! Want to know a secret?

It's all stories, you know.

Yes! Those tales we tell ourselves about what we can (and can't do), how other people make us feel, what we need to be happy.

All illusions.

And as we start to unravel these stories more and more, we start to see the simplicity in life.

Because all we ever want and need, is already here.

It's who we are.

And if not one word of this makes sense at the moment, that's ok.